One
Swing Set
Workout

Karen M. Goeller
Brian Dowd

www.SwingSetFitness.com

ISBN: 1434812596
EAN: 9781434812599

Always keep safety in mind!

Be prepared to compete with gravity during these extreme movements and exercises. You will not believe what can be done with a swing!

With many of these exercises you will not only gain strength in the specified muscle group, but additional muscle groups will become involved in order to complete the movement. You will become accustomed to supporting your own body weight.

You will be amazed at the number of exercises Karen has transferred to a swing set all because she went to the beach one day, saw a swing set, and visualized one exercise, then another, and she continued to go through several exercises.

When you see these exercises and the transition to the swing set you will amazed. These exercises are effective in targeting the muscle groups intended and the intensity of each exercise is tremendous.

Please keep in mind these exercises are not for beginners. By performing these exercises you accept the responsibility for your own personal safety and release the authors, models, and producers of this book from any liability for injuries resulting from the use of this workout and the swing set fitness books.

We hope you enjoy this workout and wish you the best of luck in reaching your fitness goals!

Safety Tips

Make sure the swing set and swing are very secure and stable. They must be in very good working condition.

Make sure you do not place your hands on glass, animal droppings, or anything that could cause you harm or illness. Sweep the area prior to use for glass or other dangerous fragments and bring a piece of foam or rubber matting for your hands and forearms.

Make sure you will not swing or bump into anyone.

Always hold the chains securely. You could lose your balance and holding the chains may help prevent a fall to the ground.

Only perform these exercises if you have discussed it with your doctor and you are healthy enough to perform strenuous and challenging exercises.

These exercises are challenging. Only perform these exercises if you are able to focus on your safety and technique. Any distractions could be dangerous.

If using a public playground, make sure it is one that allows adults without children. Make sure you follow the rules of the playground and laws in your area.

Wash hands after workout.

Wear sunscreen.

Always keep safety in mind while training!

Disclaimer

The exercises and advice contained in this book may be too difficult or dangerous for some people. Regardless of your current health status, you should consult with a qualified medical professional to ensure that the exercises and/or workouts in this book are appropriate for your fitness level. The information contained in this book is intended for individuals in good health. Proceed with great caution and at your own risk.

Any activity involving motion or height creates the possibility of accidental injury, paralysis, or death. The instructional materials are intended for use ONLY by properly trained and qualified participants under supervised conditions. Use without proper supervision or coaching could be DANGEROUS and should NOT be undertaken or permitted. Before using, KNOW YOUR LIMITATIONS and the limitations of the equipment you plan to use, including playground equipment. If in doubt always consult a qualified instructor. Always inspect equipment for loose fittings or damage and test for stability before each use.

The writers, models, and producers of this book will not be liable for injuries or consequences sustained in the use of the instructional materials, equipment used, or location.

General Fitness

There are eight exercises in this workout. Don't be fooled, the exercises are not easy and this is not a simple workout. Most of the muscle groups in your body will be engaged during this workout, especially your core muscles. This workout has been created to help the user gain and maintain a good general fitness level.

Two to three sets per exercise are recommended and 10-15 repetitions per set are appropriate for this type of workout.

Accept the challenge and let the results speak for themselves…

Always keep safety in mind!

Bulgarian Squat

Start with your back facing the swing. Lift your right foot up behind your body to place your right shin on the swing. Allow the swing to slightly move backward. Once you are balanced with your right shin on the swing, bend your left leg to perform a single leg squat. Make sure you keep your left knee in line with the hip and the toes on that side. Make sure you do not allow your knee to move forward, beyond your toes. Keep your chest up throughout the exercise.

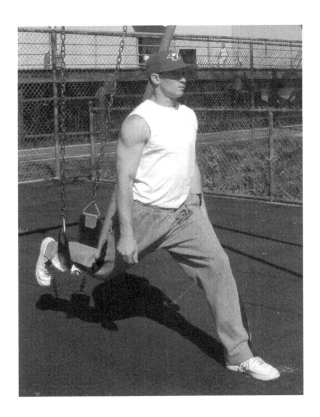

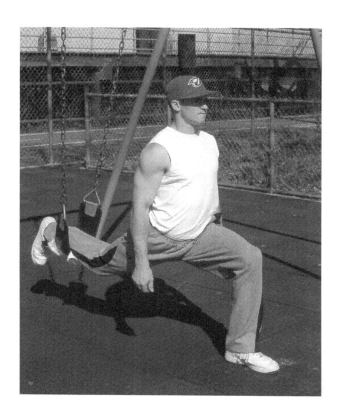

Always keep safety in mind!

Calf Raise

Start facing the swing. Grasp the center of the swing with both hands. Keeping your fingers wrapped around the bottom of the swing, walk your feet backwards so that you are at an angle. Once in position, lift your heels off the ground. Return to the starting position. Continue to lift your heels for the desired number of repetitions. Keep your chest up and your body straight throughout this exercise.

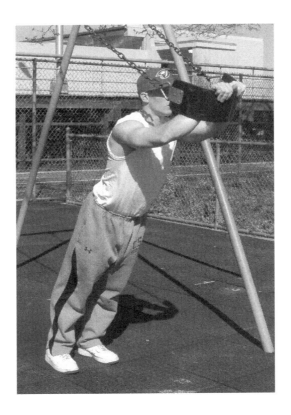

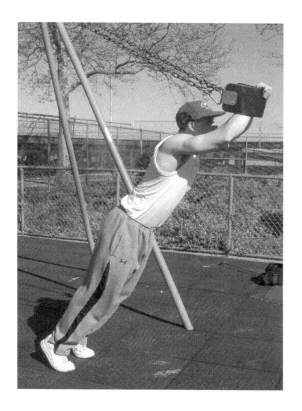

Modified Pull Up – Low

Grasp the outer portion of the swing with both hands and wrap fingers over the swing. Keeping your fingers wrapped around the bottom of the swing, lean backwards and walk your feet forward so that you are at a low position. Make sure your feet will not slide. Next, pull your chest in toward the swing. Keep your body straight throughout this exercise. You should feel this in your back and biceps.

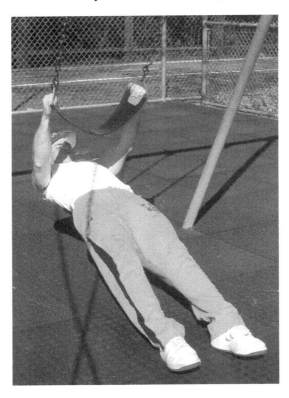

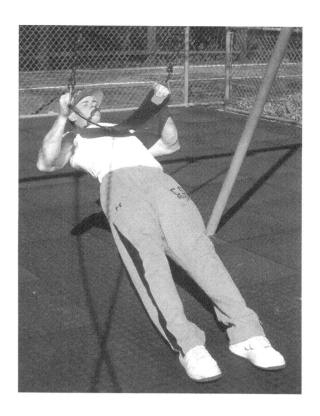

Explosive Push Ups

Start with your back facing the swing. Place your hands on the ground. Next, place your shins on the swing. You should be in a push up / plank position with your shins on the swing. Once positioned, lower your chest and chin toward the ground and then in an explosive motion, push your body up into the air. If performed correctly, your hands will leave the ground for the brief moment, because you have jumped. Make sure you bend your elbows immediately upon contact with the ground. Keep your core muscles tight and do not allow your lower back to hang down. Repeat for the desired number of repetitions. You should feel this in your chest, triceps, and core muscles.

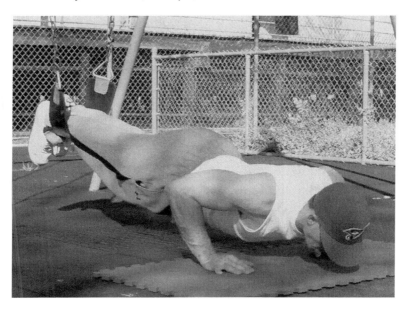

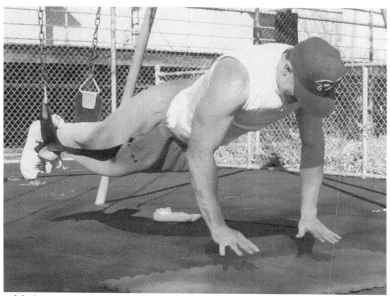

Make sure you bend your elbows immediately upon
contact with the ground.

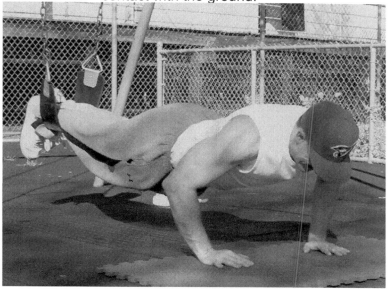

Full Pike / Virtual Handstand with Shrug

Start with your back facing the swing. Place your hands on the ground. Next, place your shins on the swing. You should be in a push up / plank position with your shins on the swing. Next, pull your belly in so that you bend at the hips to form a full pike position, virtual handstand. Your hips will be directly above your head. Your legs and arms will remain straight. Your upper body will be in a virtual handstand. Once in the virtual handstand, shrug your shoulders so that your shoulders move toward your ears. Return to the straight push up / plank position and repeat the full pike and shrug for the desired number of repetitions. You should feel this in your core, chest, and shoulder muscles.

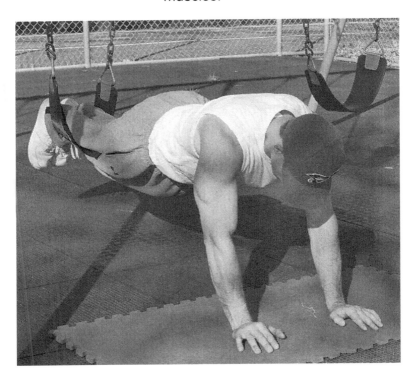

Only pull up to the full pike if you are strong enough to support your body weight upside down.

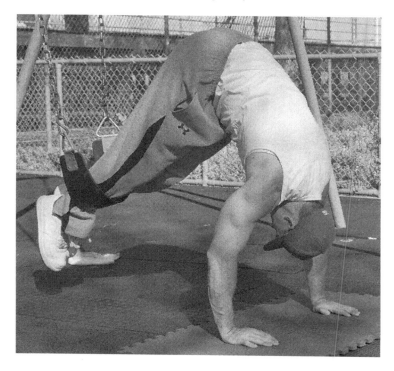

Always keep safety in mind!

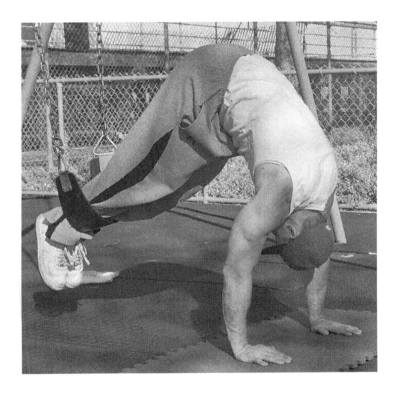

Push Up Alternate Lifts - Shins on Swing

Start with your back facing the swing. Place your hands on the ground. Next, place your shins / ankles on the swing. You should be in a push up / plank position with your shins on the swing. Lift your right hand and your left leg up simultaneously. Return your right hand to the ground and left leg to the swing then repeat the motion with your left hand and right leg. Your arms and legs remain straight. Keep your back straight and core muscles tight. Repeat the alternate lifts for the desired number of repetitions. You should feel this in your core muscles.

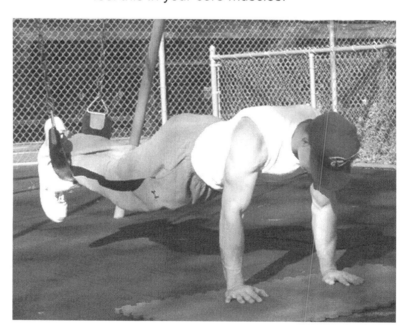

Always keep safety in mind!

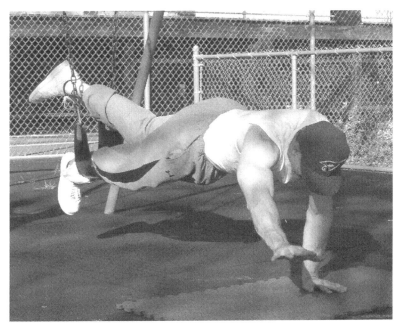

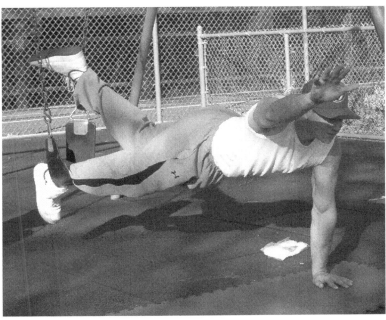

Oblique Crunch – Knees Bent

Sit on the swing, hold the chains, and lean back. Lift both legs to hip / swing height. Next, roll over toward your right hip so that your belly faces the left chain. Once both legs are bent and at hip height, lift them up and toward your left armpit. Return your legs to the starting position. Continue to perform side bent knee crunches for the desired number of repetitions. You should feel this in your side, your oblique muscles.

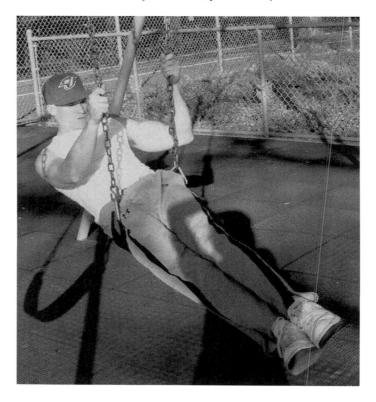

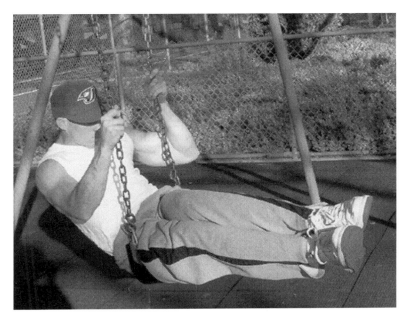

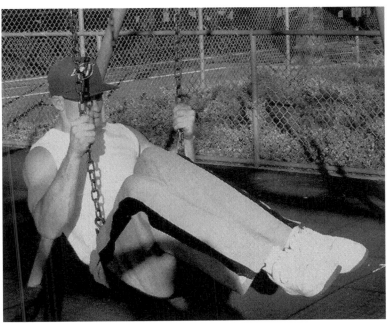

Double Crunch

Sit on the swing, hold the chains, and lean back. Lift both legs in front of your body to hip /swing height. Once both legs are at hip / swing height, bring both knees in toward your chest together. As you bring your knees in toward your chest, sit up to allow your chest and knees to meet. Once your knees and chest have formed a tuck position, return to the starting position. Continue to bring your knees in and chest up for the desired number of repetitions. You should feel this in your abdominal and hip flexor muscles.

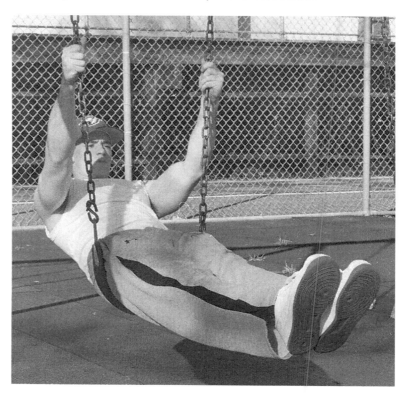

Always keep safety in mind!

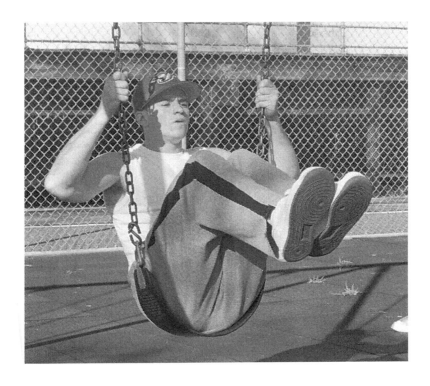

Always keep safety in mind!

About Karen Goeller

Karen Goeller's gymnastics career spans over 30 years, as a gymnast, gymnastics coach, gymnastics facility owner, and as a published author.

This amazing author has written more gymnastics books than any one person in the USA with sales worldwide. She has helped educate thousands in the gymnastics community as a coach and writer. Her books are currently used by gymnastics coaches, fitness experts, and physical education teachers among many other professionals.

Karen Goeller's published works include the famous gymnastics drills and conditioning books, gymnastics and fitness journals, a gymnastics parent's guide, and several fitness training programs.

Karen Goeller has had gymnastics articles published in USA Gymnastics Technique Magazine and on various websites. Her articles include, "The Handstand is the Most Important Skill," "Ahh...The Glide Kip," "Fun with Running, a Crucial Skill", and "Cast Handstand" among others.

Before her success as a published author, Karen Goeller owned and operated a gymnastics club in NYC for 10 years, worked for the most famous gymnastics coach, Bela Karolyi, worked at International Gymnastics Camp for a decade of holiday clinics, and worked at various health clubs in NYC.

Before she earned her BA Degree, Karen Goeller's studies included Physical Therapy, Health Sciences, Nutrition, and Emergency Medical Care. She has held certifications such as a NY State EMT, Nutritional

www.SwingSetFitness.com

Analysis, Fitness Trainer, Counseling Techniques, Childcare Fundamentals, USA Gymnastics Safety, USA Gymnastics Skill Evaluator, and USA Gymnastics Meet Director, among many others.

Besides being author to this book, Karen Goeller was one of two photographers.

Special thanks to **Steven Porter**, contributing photographer. He has captured scenic views, special moments, and action shots. Much of his work has been featured on posters, t-shirts, mugs, and other gift items sold through PortersGifts.com.

Always keep safety in mind!

Other Books by Karen Goeller

Fitness on a Swing Set
ISBN: 9780615147888

Fitness on a Swing Set with Training Programs
ISBN: 9780615150284

Swing Set Workouts
ISBN: 9780615151700

Gymnastics Drills and Conditioning Exercises
ISBN: 9781411605794

Gymnastics Drills and Conditioning for the Handstand
ISBN: 9781411650008

Gymnastics Drills: Walkover, Limber, Back Handspring
ISBN: 9781411611603

Gymnastics Conditioning for the Legs and Ankles
ISBN: 9781411620339

Gymnastics Journal: My Scores, My Goals, My Dreams
ISBN: 9781411641457

Most Frequently Asked Questions about Gymnastics
ISBN: 1591133726

Fitness Journal: Goals, Training, and Success
ISBN: 9781847284440

Strength Training Journal
ISBN: Not yet assigned.

Gymnastics Conditioning: Five Conditioning Workouts
ISBN: 9780615147598

Gymnastics Conditioning: Tumbling Conditioning
ISBN: Not yet assigned.

www.GymnasticsBooks.com

Always keep safety in mind!

About Brian Dowd

For Brian Dowd, this is his first contribution to a published work. He was the one who carefully tested more than 50 exercises to make sure they really could be transferred to a swing. That same day Brian Dowd also worked as the fitness model for this project. He posed several times for each exercise to help ensure the photo was not only captured, but that his form was technically correct.

Brian Dowd's sport has always been baseball. He has been a member of numerous travel baseball teams growing up and competed in the AAU, NABF, AABC National Championships, and the AAU Junior Olympics National Championships among others. Brian also played 4 years of varsity baseball for one of the best and most respected high school programs in New York City. After high school, Brian went on to play 4 years of NCAA College Baseball and now plays semi-professional baseball in the New York area. Brian Dowd currently coaches the high school team he once played for in New York City.

This amazing baseball player has learned a great deal about fitness and sports conditioning throughout the years and has now made a major contribution to the completion of these highly useful fitness books.

Always keep safety in mind!

Made in the USA
Charleston, SC
08 March 2010